Vandana Tendolkar

Effects of radiotherapy and chemotherapy on chromosomes

Vandana Tendolkar

Effects of radiotherapy and chemotherapy on chromosomes

LAP LAMBERT Academic Publishing

Impressum / Imprint

Bibliografische Information der Deutschen Nationalbibliothek: Die Deutsche Nationalbibliothek verzeichnet diese Publikation in der Deutschen Nationalbibliografie; detaillierte bibliografische Daten sind im Internet über http://dnb.d-nb.de abrufbar.

Alle in diesem Buch genannten Marken und Produktnamen unterliegen warenzeichen-, marken- oder patentrechtlichem Schutz bzw. sind Warenzeichen oder eingetragene Warenzeichen der jeweiligen Inhaber. Die Wiedergabe von Marken, Produktnamen, Gebrauchsnamen, Handelsnamen, Warenbezeichnungen u.s.w. in diesem Werk berechtigt auch ohne besondere Kennzeichnung nicht zu der Annahme, dass solche Namen im Sinne der Warenzeichen- und Markenschutzgesetzgebung als frei zu betrachten wären und daher von jedermann benutzt werden dürften.

Bibliographic information published by the Deutsche Nationalbibliothek: The Deutsche Nationalbibliothek lists this publication in the Deutsche Nationalbibliografie; detailed bibliographic data are available in the Internet at http://dnb.d-nb.de.

Any brand names and product names mentioned in this book are subject to trademark, brand or patent protection and are trademarks or registered trademarks of their respective holders. The use of brand names, product names, common names, trade names, product descriptions etc. even without a particular marking in this works is in no way to be construed to mean that such names may be regarded as unrestricted in respect of trademark and brand protection legislation and could thus be used by anyone.

Coverbild / Cover image: www.ingimage.com

Verlag / Publisher:
LAP LAMBERT Academic Publishing
ist ein Imprint der / is a trademark of
AV Akademikerverlag GmbH & Co. KG
Heinrich-Böcking-Str. 6-8, 66121 Saarbrücken, Deutschland / Germany
Email: info@lap-publishing.com

Herstellung: siehe letzte Seite /
Printed at: see last page
ISBN: 978-3-659-39448-5

Zugl. / Approved by: New Delhi, All India Institute of Medical Sciences, M. Sc. Dissertation, 1985

Cytogenetic Effects of Radiotherapy and Chemotherapy on Uterine Cervical and Oral Cancer Patients

This work is dedicated to those cancer patients, who in spite of their sufferings volunteered their blood samples, without which this study could not have been conducted.

Table of Contents

Introduction and Review of Literature

Over the last few decades, radiotherapy (RT) and chemotherapy (CT) are increasingly being used in the treatment of various diseases, particularly cancers. The untoward effects of these diagnostic and therapeutic maneuvers sometimes appear many years later.

RT is the use of high energy rays to stop cancer cells from growing and multiplying. Radiation destroys the ability of all cells within its reach- cancerous and normal, to grow and reproduce. However, cancer cells are more sensitive to radiation than normal cells. X-rays and gamma rays are the commonest form of therapeutic radiation. The mode and amount of radiation used to treat the variety of known human cancers is highly variable. Although the harmful effects of radiation exposure have been recognized for quite some time now, the full impact of these effects has yet to be elucidated completely. The intricacies of tissue vulnerability, age of the patient, type of radiation and dosage, other accompanying therapies (such as CT) and the underlying disease complicate the precise evaluation of the risks and benefits.

Chemotherapeutic drugs used for the treatment of cancers are basically cytotoxic or cytostatic in their effects. That is, they reduce cell division, or cause cell death. Both these effects are brought about via interaction with the genetic material. Some of these drugs are known to be toxic and mutagenic to normal tissues, particularly the rapidly proliferating ones, viz. hemopoietic tissue. Some drugs have been shown to be carcinogenic as well.

Ever since RT and CT were implemented in the treatment of cancers, their mutagenicity had been suspected. The analysis of chromosome damage in persons exposed to exceptionally high levels of chemicals, and x-rays or gamma rays became the area of interest as soon as improved methods for chromosomal analysis became available.

Conen (1961) was the first to report chromosome damage following cytostatic therapy. Ryan et al (1965) found that in patients treated with methotrexate, the cultured peripheral blood lymphocytes showed chromosome gaps and breaks more commonly in chromosomes 1 and 3. There are reports of induction of polyploidy and endoreduplication (Nasjleti et al, 1965), of breakage and aberrations (Kawasaki et al, 1966) and of dicentrics, rings and long chromosomes, acentric fragments and chromosomal exchanges (Kawasaki et al, 1967) following treatment of patients with various cytotoxic drugs.

Warren et al (1965) reported chromosomal analysis in patients of lung and cervical cancer, before, during and after RT. Before RT, they were normal and at low doses, hypodiploidy was common. However, with higher doses they reported chromosome fragments, dicentrics and atypical configurations. At doses of about 8,410 rads, ring chromosomes were seen. They also mentioned that the relative frequency of different aberration types becomes less with increasing time period after the irradiation. However, atypical chromosomes were occasionally seen as long as 30 years later. This is in accordance with Tough's (1960) earlier findings.

In more recent times, Riguad et al (1990) have reported chromosomal aberrations in circulating lymphocytes induced by RT and CT. They studied serially collected blood samples before and after RT and CT and combined treatments. They found that local RT induced unstable chromosome aberrations. Dicentrics were the most common finding, with a time-dependent decrease in frequency. In a similar study, Legal et al (2002) found that the rate of stable chromosomal aberrations increased significantly after RT, and persisted at least for a year thereafter. Chromosome and chromatid aberrations following RT were reported by Vinnikov et al (2010) also.

Mutational events in normal tissues, induced by RT and/ or CT of a primary neoplasm may cause their transformation to malignant tissue, giving rise to secondary neoplasia in patients who are successfully treated for a primary neoplasm. Yet the benefits derived from therapeutic irradiation for many malignancies far outweigh the potential risks. In fact, in many instances, it is the prolongation of survival and achievement of a near normal life, due to radiation therapy which has simultaneously allowed the patient to be at an increased risk of malignancy in later life.

Routine mutagenicity testing, if done on patients receiving RT and CT, would be of great value in identifying individuals with increased genetic and/or cancer risk, for establishing safe levels of exposure, and for protection of human society as a whole.

Materials and Methods

Selection of patients

Cancer patients were selected to study the effect of radiotherapy and /or chemotherapy on chromosomes of peripheral blood lymphocytes. Oral (tongue, cheek and soft palate) and uterine cervical cancer patients were preferred owing to the high incidence of these two types of cancers in India. Blood samples were collected from patients registered with Radiotherapy Department of Sufdarjung Hospital, for treatment. Samples were drawn with voluntary consent of patients. Clinical history was recorded from the patients' file and family history was recorded by interviewing the patient and his/her relatives.

All the cases included in this study had undergone biopsy. Histopathological findings of the biopsy material confirmed them as cases of primary malignancies. Cases with any type of pre-treatment exposure to therapeutic irradiation/chemotherapy were excluded. Some patients had undergone surgery and were on radiotherapy.

Patients were interviewed at their first visit to the Radiotherapy Department. For uterine cervical cancer patients emphasis was given to record their marital status and sexual habits. In case of oral cancer patients importance was given to record their quid-chewing, smoking and drinking habits. Pre-treatment samples were drawn on that day. Later, during the course of RT/CT, blood samples were collected at various intervals, ranging from the 5th day of the onset of therapy to the 30th day. During the follow-up visits by the patients post-treatment blood samples were collected.

In all, 60 patients were investigated. Of these 14 were oral cancer patients (8 Ca tongue, 4 Ca cheek and 2 Ca palate); three of them were on CT courses after having been exposed to unsuccessful RT doses of 6,500 rads, 4,500 rads and 5,800 rads. The former two were Ca tongue patients and the latter Ca cheek.

The remaining 46 patients were diagnosed as having uterine cervical cancer in various clinical stages. Staging for uterine cervical carcinoma was done on the basis of the following standard criteria.

Pre-invasive carcinoma

- Stage 0   Carcinoma in situ; intra-epithelial carcinoma.

Invasive carcinoma

- Stage I   Carcinoma strictly confined to the cervix
- Stage II   The carcinoma extends beyond the cervix, but has not extended on the pelvic wall. The carcinoma involves the vagina, but not the lower third.
- Stage III   The carcinoma has extended on to the pelvic wall. On rectal examination there is no cancer-free space between the tumor and the pelvic wall. The tumor involves the lower third of the vagina. All cases with a hydronephrosis or non-functioning kidney should be included unless they are known to be due to other cause.

- Stage IV   The carcinoma has extended beyond the true pelvis or has clinically involved the mucosa of the bladder or rectum.

Among the 46 cervical cancer patients included in this study, 4 were diagnosed as Stage I patients, 19 as Stage II, and 23 as Stage III patients. Two of the patients in Stage II, and one in Stage III had undergone surgical treatment before palliative RT was recommended. Cervical cancer patients were of 28 to 65 years and oral cancer patients were of 40 to 74 years of age.

The patients belonged to various income groups. Most of those with cervical cancer came from the category of daily wage laborers, *jamadars* and sweepers. However, almost 50% of oral cancer patients were educated and belonged to middle income group families.

None of the patients had a family history of any type of cancer. Also, the patients themselves had no other apparent clinical abnormality, any disease or obvious genetic abnormality which might be a predisposing factor in the occurrence of the oral/cervical cancer. All the patients suffering from uterine cervical cancer were married and had given birth to two or more children, except Case VIII. Smoking, particularly tobacco smoking, *paan* and tobacco quid chewing, non-vegetarian diet and alcohol consumption are well-known pre-disposing factors in the occurrence of oral cancers; therefore the incidence of these habits among oral cancer patients were taken special note of.

Normal subjects and untreated patients suffering from oral and cervical cancer served as controls for the study.

Methodology

Peripheral blood samples were collected from the patients personally. Lymphocyte cultures were set up. Chromosome preparations were stained with conventional stains, and for G and C banding.

I: <u>Blood lymphocyte culture technique</u>

1. 5ml of peripheral blood was drawn in a heparinized syringe and allowed to stand for 2 hours at 37° C.
2. With gentle tapping of the syringe 0.5-1.0 ml of plasma containing cells was added to the culture bottle containing 5ml of TC 199+0.2ml phytohemagluttinin.
3. Cultures were incubated for 72 hours at 37° C and were gently shaken twice a day.
4. After 70 hours of incubation, 0.1ml of colcemid (0.02 mg/ml) was added to the cultures.
5. At 72 hours the cultures were transferred to centrifuge tubes and centrifuged at 1000rpm for 10 minutes.
6. Supernatant was discarded and the cells were resuspended in 5ml of pre-warmed KCl (0.56%). Cells were incubated for 10 minutes and were centrifuged again.
7. Supernatant was discarded and the cells fixed in 5-7ml of fixative (methanol+glacial acetic acid, 3:1) for 30 minutes at room   temperature.
8. Two to three changes of fixative were given.
9. Few drops of cell suspension were dropped on a wet, clean slide and dried vigorously.

10. For conventional staining, slides were stained in 4% Giemsa.Slides were mounted in DPX using 24X40mm cover slips. Free end of slide was labeled.

II. G-Banding Technique

A modified technique of Seabright (1971) was used, which is as follows:

1. Unstained chromosomal preparations were treated with 0.25% trypsin (Difco) in an isotonic solution for 1-2 minutes.
2. Slides were stained in 4% Giemsa at pH 6.8 for 5-7 minutes.
3. Slides were washed in running tap water, dried and mounted in DPX.

III. C-Banding Technique

A modified technique of Sumner (1972) was used, which is as follows:

1. Unstained chromosome preparations were treated with 0.2N hydrochloric acid at room temperature for 45 minutes.
2. Slides were rinsed in distilled water.
3. Slides were incubated in 5% barium hydroxide solution at 56° C for 15 minutes.
4. Slides were thoroughly washed in distilled water to remove all traces of barium hydroxide.
5. Slides were then incubated in SSC* (0.3 M sodium chloride + 0.03 M trisodium citrate) solution at 60° C for one hour.
6. Slides were washed in distilled water.
7. Slides were stained in 4% Giemsa, pH 6.8, for 5-7 minutes.

8. Excess stain was washed in distilled water, the slides dried and examined under the microscope.

*To prepare 2SSC solution, dissolve 17.538 grams sodium chloride and 8.82 grams trisodium citrate in one liter distilled water.

IV. Photomicrography

Selected metaphase spreads were photographed on Carl Zeiss photomicroscope using a slow NP 15 film. Exposed films were developed and fixed according to standard procedures. Photographic prints were made on Agfa Brovira 'Special' grade paper. Prints were exposed for approximately 10 seconds and were developed and fixed according to standard procedures.

Karyotypes of selected metaphase spreads were prepared by cutting and pairing the chromosomes.

Results and Discussion

Cancer of Uterine Cervix (Ca Cx)

Etiologic Factors

Most of the patients were in the age group of 35-45 years (Table 1). All patients except one had been married around the age of menarche, and had first coitus before age 16, and were mothers before 20 years of age. It appears that age at first coitus and early motherhood may increase the risk for Ca Cx.

The importance of age at first coitus may derive from the susceptibility of the adolescent cervix to atypical transformations. In India, where girls generally get married at a young age, and bear multiple children, these may be factors contributing to the high incidence of this type of cancer. Wahi, et al (1972) also suggested early marriage, early coitus, and multiparity to be of some etiologic significance.

Table 1: Age Incidence and Clinical Stages of Cancer of Uterine Cervix

Age Group (Years)	No. of Patients	No. of Patients in Clinical Stages		
		I	II	III
25-35	6	-	2	4
35-45	17	2	8	7
45-55	16	2	6	8
55-65	7	-	3	4

As has been stated earlier, cases included in this study came from one of the largest general hospitals in Delhi. Almost all of them belonged to rather low income group. Whether there is any correlation between socio-economic background and incidence of Ca Cx is difficult to document. However, in low income group, marriages tend to take place at an early age and have a large number of children (due to lack of use of contraception). Early marriage and large number of children may be responsible for the higher incidence of Ca Cx.

Related to socio-economic class is another etiologic factor of importance- the availability of clean water and penile hygiene. Wakefield, et al (1973) suggested an association between socio-economic group and incidence of Ca Cx though no substantial data are available.

Most patients attending the radiotherapy clinic came from nearby villages and suburbs. Due to financial constraints and lack of adequate health facilities, several months pass from the time the disease becomes clinically manifest, diagnosed and finally treated at this hospital. This perhaps is the reason for finding (Table 1) most of the cases in clinical stages II and III (well-advanced stages). Obviously, the prognosis of these patients gets poor.

Cytogenetic Findings

I. Radiotherapy

Of the 46 Ca Cx patients studied, 18 belonged to pre-treatment group, 18 to on-treatment group, and 10 to post-treatment (7 post-radiotherapy, 3 post-radiotherapy and post-chemotherapy) group. Of these metaphases could be analyzed from 7 pre-treatment, 3 on-treatment and 2 post-treatment samples. An average of 16.5 metaphases was scored from each case (Table 2 & 3).

Normal chromosome count of 46 was seen in 12.2 metaphases from untreated, 2.0 from on-treatment and in 6.0 from post-treatment samples.

➢ Untreated samples

The high incidence of hypomodal cells in untreated samples (Table 2) may be attributed partly to technical errors. In the on-treatment samples, hypomodal cells were four times more numerous than the hypermodal cells (Table 2). The chromosome loss was random, which may be due to an effect of radiation beams hitting the mitotic apparatus.

The average number of hyperdiploid metaphases was 0.8 in the untreated group, 2.0 in the on-treatment group and 2.5 in the post-treatment group (Table 2). The increase in frequency of hyperdiploid cells may be due to radiation-induced partial duplication of chromosomes. During RT there may be some degree of mitotic suppression. After cessation of radiation exposure the affected cells enter mitosis, whereupon the hyperdiploidy becomes evident. However, the difference in percentage of hyperdiploid cells between the on-treatment and post-treatment cases has to be over-looked at present, since the sample size is small.

Table 2: Chromosome Counts in Various Groups

S. No.	Groups	Average no. of metaphases with chromosomal counts		
		39-45	46	47-50
1.	Normal/Pretreatment	3.0	12.1	0.8
2.	On-treatment	5.0	2.0	2.0
3.	Post-treatment	8.0	6.0	2.5

Table 3: Incidence of Chromosomal Aberrations in Pre-treatment Samples and Its Co-relation   with Age and Clinical Stage of the Patient

S. No.	Age (Years)	Stage of Cancer	Total No. of Metaphases	Metaphases With			
				Chromosome Counts			Structural Aberrations
				39-45	46	47-50	
1-5	25-40	Normal	12	-	12	-	-
Case I	28	II	7	3	4	-	-
Case II	40	II	20	2	8	8	-
Case III	40	III	25	4	20	1	2; gap & DMB
Case IV	42	I	5	1	4	-	-
Case V	60	II	11	6	5	-	-
Case VI	50	I	3	2	1	-	-
Case VII	40	II	58	9	48	1	-

Numerical chromosomal abnormalities are termed as aneuploidy. A chromosomal count of less than 46 is hypodiploidy; more than 46 is hyperdiploidy. Aneuploidy may be due to increased chromosome fragility and may be an important factor in the development of malignant conditions. The genetic imbalance provides a possible reason for an increase of spontaneous malfunction of the cellular system, as well as for an increased sensitivity to external factors.

G-banding (Fig. 2 & 3) and C-banding (Fig. 4) were done in untreated cancer patients and non-cancerous subjects (Fig. 1). Cases I, III and VI from the untreated group were followed up during treatment (Table 4).

Fig. 1. Metaphase spread from Case I, untreated sample 46,XX.

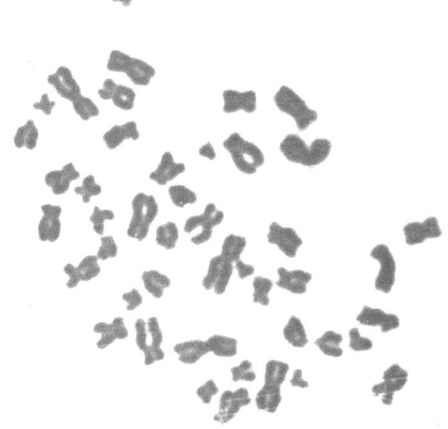

Fig. 2. G-banded metaphase spread; Case VII, untreated sample.

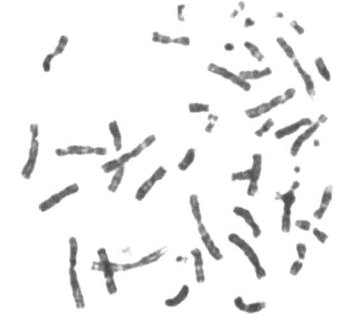

Fig. 3. G-banded karyotypes, Case VII; prepared from metaphase spread shown in Fig. 2. 46, XX.

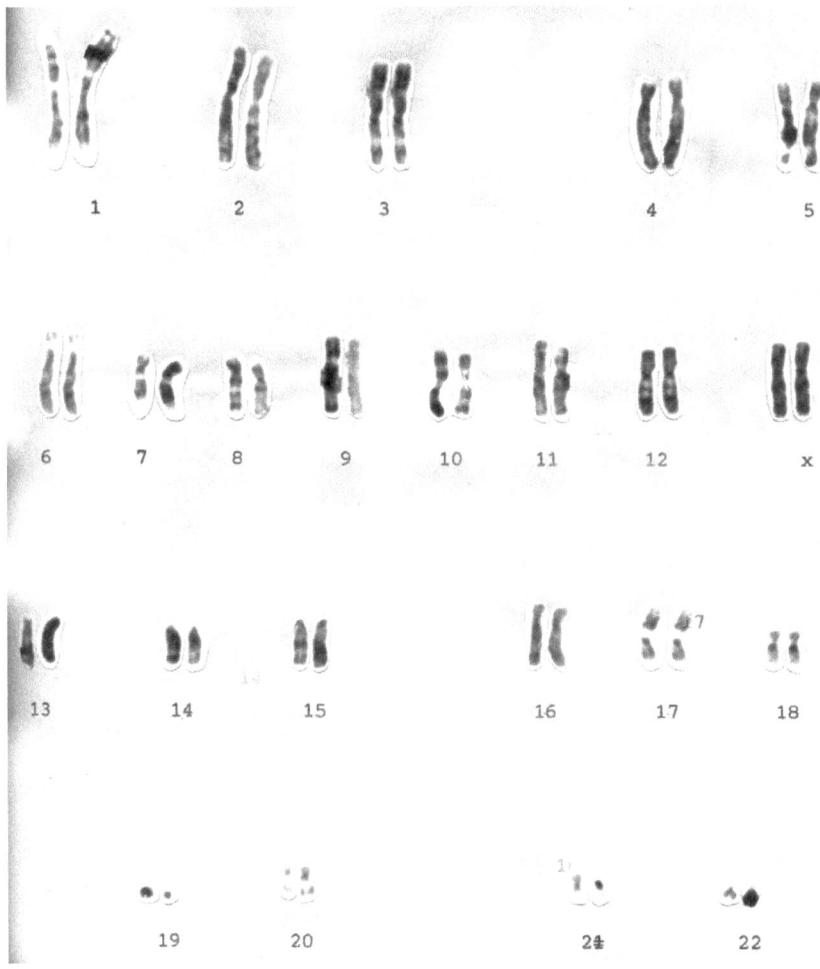

Fig. 4. C-banded metaphase spread from non-cancerous subject.

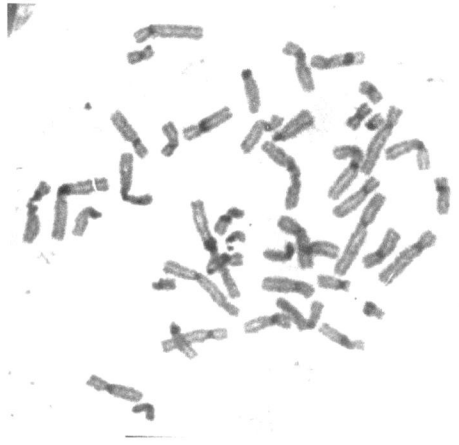

Table 4: Incidence of Chromosomal Aberrations in On-Treatment Samples from Uterine Cervical Cancer Patients

S. No.	Age (Years)	Stage of Cancer	RT Exposure Dose (Rads)	Total No. of Metaphases	Metaphases With			
					Chromosome Counts			Structural Aberrations
					39-45	46	47-50	
Case I	28	II	5,510	26	19	3	4	4 isochromatid breaks, 2 dicentrics, 3 pulverized metaphases
Case III	40	III	213	7	2	3	2	-
Case IV	50	I	663	4	3	1	-	-

> On-treatment samples

Chromosome damage following exposure to radiation was seen in case I (Figures 5 & 6). This patient, in clinical stage II, had been exposed to 5,510 rads over a period of 6 weeks.

Fig. 5. A metaphase spread from Case I, on-treatment sample, showing pulverization of chromosomes after exposure to 5,510 rads.

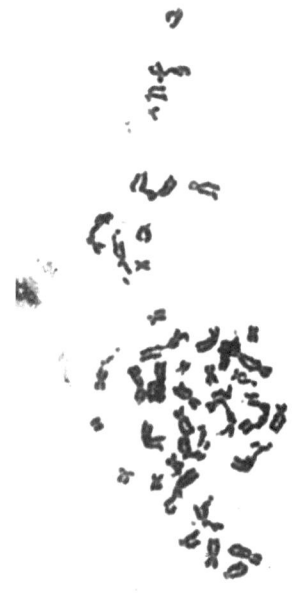

Four of twenty-six metaphases analyzed showed structural chromosomal abnormalities like an isochromatid break, two dicentrics, and three pulverized metaphases. The pulverized metaphases depicted breaks of the chromatid type (Figure 5), i.e. break in only one chromosome arm. This kind of break must have occurred following DNA replication in the cell cycle.

Chromosome damage is a common aftermath of irradiation. Fate of broken chromosomes depends much up on the site of the break. A break not affecting the centromere produces a shorter chromosome with a centromere and an acentric fragment. This acentric fragment (Figure 5) runs a high risk of being lost during the subsequent mitosis.

Chromosomes broken at two breaking points may rejoin under the influence of repair enzymes, or may join with break points from other chromosomes, homologous or non-homologous. The random breaking and rejoining may result in various types of chromosomal rearrangements.

Two dicentrics were seen in a metaphase from case I (Figure 6).

Fig. 6. Metaphase spread, Case I, on treatment, showing two dicentrics and one isochromatid break after exposure to 5,510 rads.

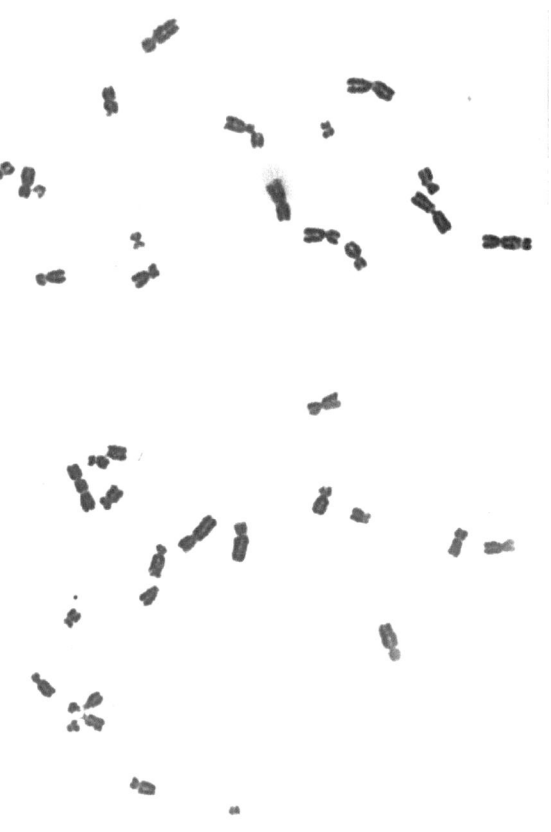

Dicentrics is a common finding in blood samples from irradiated individuals. Dicentrics are formed by chromosome breakage and joining between different chromosomes, homologous or non-homologous. If breakage occurs in G1 phase, joining follows in the G1 (or early S) phase before DNA replication. If each of the broken chromosomes happens to have one centromere, the translocated chromosome will have two centromeres and may pass through the next mitosis without difficulty under the following conditions:

(1)   The centromeres migrate to the same poles, and

(2)   Replication and sister chromatid exchange between the two centromeres has not led to intertwining of the two chromatids.

Of the 26 metaphases analyzed in case I, only 3 were normal (Table 4); 19 were hypomodal (Figures 7 and 8). Case VI also showed 75% metaphases with hypomodal number. There was a random loss of chromosomes in all these cases. Such an increase in number of hypomodal cells cannot be entirely attributed to irradiation; it could partly be due to technical errors. To support the finding of increased number of cells with hypomodal chromosomes, more cases and metaphases need to be analyzed.

Fig. 7. Metaphase spread, Case I, on treatment, showing an acentric fragment and an abnormal D group (13-15) chromosome, after exposure to 5,510 rads.

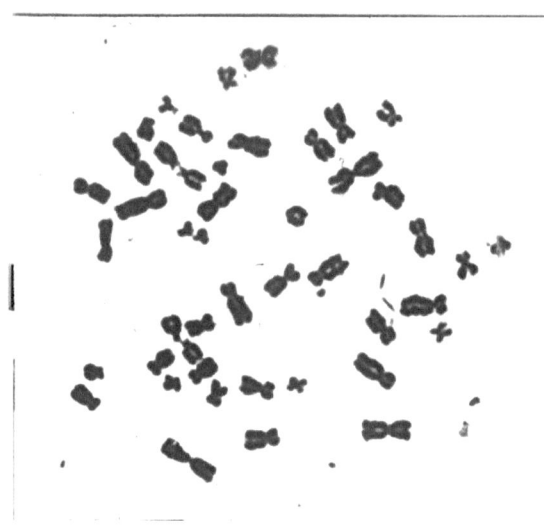

Fig. 8. Karyotype prepared from metaphase spread shown in Fig 8, Case I, exposed to 5,510 rads.

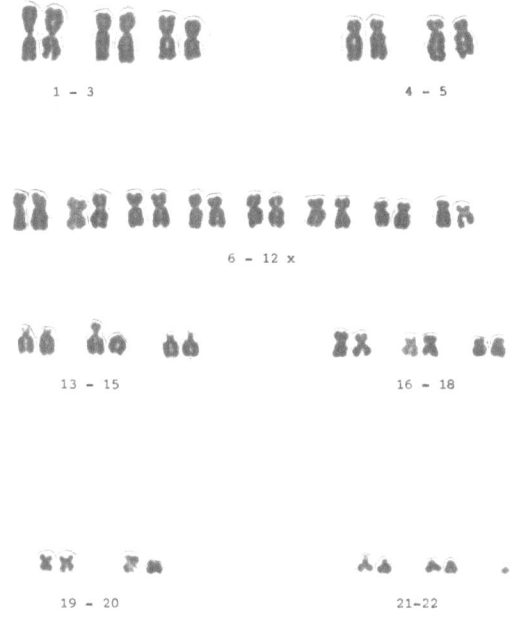

Cases IV and VIII were followed up for post-radiotherapy samples (Table 5).

Table 5: Incidence of Chromosomal Aberrations in Post-Treatment Samples from Uterine Cervical Cancer Patients

S. No.	Age (Years)	Stage of Cancer	RT Exposure Dose (Rads)	Total No. of Metaphases	Metaphases With			Structural Aberrations
					Chromosome Counts			
					39-45	46	47-50	
Case VIII	31	III	4,906	25	9	11	5	isochromatid breaks, endoreduplication, 11 dicentrics, one abnormally long chromosome with multiple centromeres, 3 pairs of DMB
Case IV	42	I	4,950	4	1	2	-	2 dicentrics

Both the patients had been exposed to 4,900 rads over a short span of four weeks. Chromosome analysis from case VIII, four weeks post-irradiation revealed in all, eleven dicentrics, one abnormally long chromosome with multiple centromeres, three pairs of double minute body (DMS), multiple isochromatid breaks (Figure 9) and endoreduplication (Figure 10).

Fig. 9. Metaphase spread, Case VIII; four weeks after exposure to 4,900 rads.

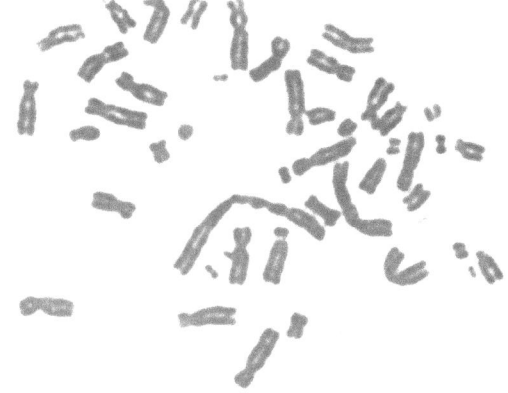

Fig.10: Metaphase spread showing endoreduplication; case VIII, four weeks after exposure to 4,900 rads

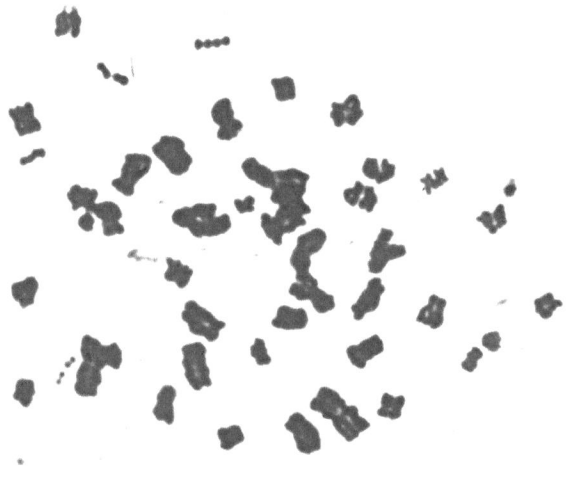

Case IV was studied eight weeks after completion of radiotherapy course. Four metaphases could be analyzed; of these, one showed two dicentric chromosomes. Mitotic counts in samples from on-treatment and post-treatment were low. Good quality G-banding, as is required to confirm structural rearrangements and aberrations could not be seen.

Endoreduplication can sometimes be seen in samples from normal subjects as well and hence cannot be taken as an effect of radiotherapy. Besides, cells from cancer patients are known to show such cell division defects.

Noteworthy, however, is the appearance of a large number of structural aberrations in post-treatment samples in contrast to numerical aberrations (hypodiploidy) in non-treatment samples. Hypodiploidy was seen in 31% metaphases analyzed in post-treatment samples, in contrast to 66% hypodiploid metaphases in the on-treatment samples. Results clearly show that different mechanisms are involved in the induction and elimination of cells with numerical and structural aberrations during the cell cycle. Owing to the time limit allowed for this study, patients could not be followed up for longer duration. Warren et al (1965) have observed cells with atypical chromosomes even after 30 years of radiotherapy. They also suggested that the aneuploidy is a transitory finding and is probably due to an effect of irradiation on the mitotic apparatus of dividing cells rather than any direct effect on the chromosomes themselves. On the other hand, structural aberrations would result from direct effect on chromosomes before a cell enters division. Many stem cells would get affected *in situ* during interphase and would thus contribute to the observed dose-dependent increase in frequency of cells with structural aberrations; successive bombardment of the lymphopoietic tissue by the x-ray beam would then compound the pre-existing injury giving rise to the multiple breakage which characterizes the chromosome picture late in the course of therapy and in the early months thereafter.

A number of samples drawn from the on-treatment and post-treatment group could not be analyzed owing to poor cell growth *in vitro*. Also, there were multiple drop-outs, either due to side-effects of radiotherapy and poor prognosis, or on clinician's advice for termination of RT before completion of prescribed dose.

Attempts were made to confirm the abnormal/multiple centromere positions by de-staining the conventionally stained slides and re-staining for C-banding. Chromosome preparations were old and did not give much information.

II. Chemotherapy

Blood samples were analyzed from three patients in clinical stage III after having intravenous injections (Table 6). Two of them had received prior radiotherapy (8,000 and 9,500 rads) but the tumor had failed to respond.

Table 6: Amount of Radiotherapy and Types of Chemotherapeutic Drugs Administered to Cervical Cancer Patients

Case No.	Clinical stage	History of Radiotherapy	Chemotherapy
XXIII	III	No History	1. Methotrexate 105mg 2. Endoxan 1600mg
XXIV	III	6,500 rads in 1982 3,000 rads in 1984	Blood sample drawn 4 weeks after I/V inj of: 1. Vincristine 1mg 2. Bleomycin 12mg 3. Mitomycin C 40mg
XXV	IIb	8,100 rads	1. Vincristine 2mg 2. Bleomycin 24mg 3. Mitomycin C 40mg
XXVI	III	6,500 rads in 1982 1,500 rads in 1983	Endoxan 1200mg

Lymphocyte cultures from patients on radiotherapy and chemotherapy showed poor cell growth and un-analyzable metaphases. This was probably the effect of cytostatic drugs on the cells and cell division. Gebhart et al (1980) reported similar experience. However, they could analyze some metaphases with chromosomal aberrations after treatment with 5-flurouracil and vincristine.

Cancers of the Oral Cavity

Etiologic Factors

Fifty-three per cent of the patients studied were in the age group of 50-60. There appears to be an increase in incidence of oral cancers from age 40 onwards. Rarely patients of less than 30 or 35 years of age with oral cancer are seen. Although most people are heavy smokers and quid chewers in the second decade of their life, clinically overt disease appears only decades later. However, once the tumor appears, it is rapid in its growth and metastasis, and early death is the most common result. Cutler et al (1975) also reported steady increase in incidence of oral cancers from age 45 onwards.

Up on interviewing, it was found that twelve of the fourteen patients studied were smokers, having smoked as many as 50 cigarettes/*beedies* per day for the last thirty to forty year. This suggests a very good correlation between smoking and oral cancer incidence. In fact, Wynder and Stellman (1977) reported a four to fifteen times greater risk for oral cancer for cigarette smokers.

Fifty per cent of the patients were, or had been *paan* or tobacco quid chewers. The sample size being small, it is not possible to state that *paan* or tobacco chewing greatly increases oral cancer incidence. However, studies on larger populations by other workers (Simarak et al, 1977) do suggest a positive correlation.

Fifty seven per cent cases were also moderate drinkers. It is difficult to say how far alcohol consumption by itself contributes to risk of oral cancer, since alcoholics were smokers also. In 1982, Schottenfield et al have reported that the risk of oral cancer for heavy drinkers in combination with tobacco is approximately seven times greater than that of non-smokers and non-alcoholics. A multiplicative or synergistic effect has been suggested for alcohol and tobacco smoking, with risk for combined exposure being greater than the additive effects of each factor (Wynder et al, 1977).

Most of these cases with habit of *paan* chewing, smoking and drinking were non-vegetarian also. Perhaps the longer duration of time for which this kind of food has to be chewed, or certain flavors may be acting as a tumor-promoting factor. However, this study must be done on a large scale by taking into consideration several other factors before conclusively stating positive relation between non-vegetarian diet and oral cancer incidence.

As stated earlier, patients for this study were selected from a general hospital. Hence, majority of patients belonged to low-income groups, with low education standards. Hirayama (1969) and Wynder et al (1977) reported that poor oral hygiene and indiscriminate smoking and drinking are the results of lack of education and low income, which probably increases the chances for oral cancer.

Cytogenetic Findings

I.   Radiotherapy

Of the fourteen oral cancer patients studied, 5 belonged to pre-treatment group, 6 to on-treatment group and 3 to post-treatment group. All patients in post-treatment group were on chemotherapy. Each of the five pre-treatment cases and three of the on-treatment cases showed analyzable metaphases. Blood cultures from post-radiotherapy cases showed poor growth.

➢   Untreated samples

From the five pre-treatment cases, an average of 30 metaphases was analyzed. An average of seven was hypomodal, twenty had normal counts (Figure 11) and three were hypermodal.

Fig. 11: A metaphase spread from pre-treatment sample of case XXII, showing 46, XY pattern.

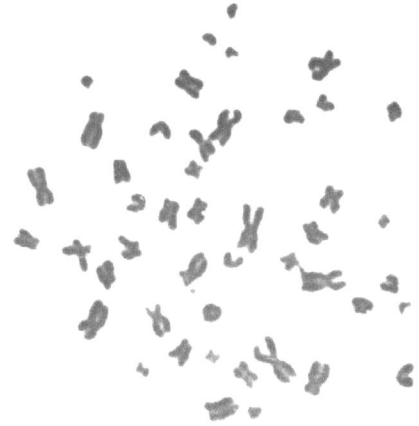

Four of the five pre-treatment samples showed structural aberration (Table 7) on an average of two metaphases each. The aberrations consisted of one chromatid break, three chromosome breaks, one dicentric, three double minute bodies, and one endoreduplicating cell.

Table 7: Incidence of Chromosomal Aberrations in Pre-treatment Samples from Oral Cancer Patients

S. No.	Age (Years); Sex	Total No. of Metaphases	Total No. of Metaphases			
			Chromosome Counts			Structural Aberrations
			39-45	46	47-50	
Case XVII	85, F	26	8	13	3	Chromatid break, DMB, pulverization
Case XIX	68, M	25	3	20	2	DMB
Case XXII	40, M	73	16	54	3	3 chromosome breaks, 1 dicentric
Case XVI	40, M	12	4	4	4	Endoreduplication, DMB
Case XVIII	55, M	15	4	8	3	-

These patients were at advanced stages of tumor progression and had swollen cervical lymph nodes. There is a large probability that the cells showing these structural chromosomal aberrations may be metastatic cells in peripheral blood.

➢ On-treatment samples

In the on-treatment group, three patients were followed (Table 8). From each, an average of 18 metaphases was analyzed. Of these, ten cells were hypomodal, five were normal and two were hypermodal.

Table 8: Incidence of Chromosomal Aberrations in Pre-treatment Samples from Oral Cancer Patients

S. No.	Age (Years); Sex	RT Exposure Dose (Rads)	Total No. of Metaphases	Total No. of Metaphases			
				Chromosome Counts			Structural Aberrations
				39-45	46	47-50	
Case XVII	85, F	1085	22	10	11	1	-
Case XIX	69, M	8858	6	3	2	1	Pulverization, DMB
Case XVIII	55, M	6,250	28	18	4	1	Isochromatid break, 2 dicentrics, 2 pulverized metaphases

Two of these on-treatment cases showed structural chromosomal aberrations. From case XIX, six metaphases could be examined, of which two showed structural aberrations, one double minute body and a pulverized metaphase (Figure 12). This patient had been exposed to 6,250 rads over a span of six weeks.

Fig. 12: A metaphase spread showing more than 73 chromosomes; case XIX, after exposure to 6,858 rads

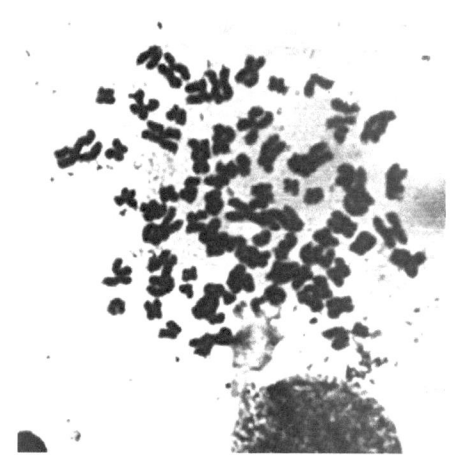

> Post-treatment samples

None of the patients could be followed-up for post-therapy samples for various reasons. The patients showed poor prognosis, the radiotherapy was thus terminated, or the patients stopped attending the clinic. The patients came from distant places and it was not feasible to follow them.

II.   Chemotherapy

Blood samples from three oral cancer patients (Table 9) on chemotherapy schedules were collected. These patients had already been on high doses of radiotherapy without much success. Blood cultures from these patients showed poor cell growth.

Table 9: Amount of Radiotherapy and Types of Chemotherapeutic Drugs Administered to Oral Cancer Patients

Case No.	Clinical Diagnosis	History of Radiotherapy	Chemotherapy
XV	Ca cheek	7,220 rads	Blood sample drawn 45 days after I/V inj of: 1. Ciplatinum 1000mg
XX	Ca, base of tongue	4,500 rads	1. Cyclophosphamide 4,500 mg 2. Vincristine 1200 mg
XXI	Ca tongue	4,000 rads	1. Cyclophosphamide 200 mg 2. Bleomycin 150 mg

Conclusions

1. Radiotherapy in high doses induces chromosomal aberrations.
2. Numerical aberrations- hypodiploid cells appear early in the course of therapy.
3. Number of hypodiploid cells reduces in post-irradiation samples.
4. In the post-irradiation samples, structural chromosomal aberrations are seen.
5. Early coitus and multiple child births predispose a woman to the cancer of uterine cervix.
6. Beedi/cigarette smoking predisposes the smoker to cancers of the oral cavity.
7. Routine chromosome analysis of irradiated samples is recommended to check
    - Secondary neoplasias, and
    - Birth of congenitally malformed babies.

Appendix I

I. Developing of photographic films

Developer for NP 15 film:

Metol   2.0gm

Hydroquinone   5.0gm

Sodium sulphite   10.0gm

Borax   2.0gm

Water   to make 1000ml

Time   7-11 minutes

Fixer:

20% Hypo (Sodium thiosulphate)

0.2% Potassium metabisulphite

II. Preparation of photographic prints

Developer for special grade paper:

Metol   1.0gm

Sodium sulphite   13.0gm

Hydroquinone   3.0gm

Sodium carbonate   26.0gm

Potassium bromide 1.0gm

Dissolve in water in given sequence

Make volume up to 1000ml

Fixer:

20% Hypo (Sodium thiosulphate)

0.2% Potassium metabisulphite

Bibliography

1. Conen, P. E. and Lansky, G. K. (1961): Chromosome damage during nitrogen mustard therapy. British medical Journal: 1961 II, 1055.

2. Gebhart, E., Losing, J. and Wopfner, F. (1980): Chromosome studies on lymphocytes of patients under cytostatic therapy. I. Conventional studies in cytostatic interval therapy. Human Genetics 55(1): 53.Cutler, S.J. and Young, J.L. Jr. (1975): Third National Cancer Survey: Incidence data. National Cancer Institute Monogram 41: 1.

3. Hirayama, T. (1966): An epidemiological study of oral and pharyngeal cancers in Central and South East Asia. Bulletin of World Health Organization 34: 41.

4. Kawasaki, M., Tojo, S., Nishimura, T. and Sugahara, T. (1966): Effect of endoxan therapy on human chromosomes. Japanese Journal of Obstetrical and Gynecological Society 13:103.

5. Nasjleti, C. E., Walden, J. M. and Spencer, H. H. (1965): Polyploidy and endoreduplication induced *in vivo* and *in vitro* in human leucocytes with N, N^1-bis (8-bromopropionyl) piperazine (A-8103). Cancer Research 25: 275.

6. Rigaud, O., Guedeney, G., Duranton, I., Leroy, A. Doloy, M. T. andMagdelenat, H. (1990): Genotoxic effects of radiotherapy and chemotherapy on the circulating lymphocytes of breast cancer patients. I. Chromosome aberrations induced *in vivo*. Mutation Research Sep; 242 (1): 17-23.

7. Ryan, T. J., Boddington, M. M. and Spriggs, A. I. (1965): Chromosome abnormalities produced by folic acid antagonists. British Journal of Dermatology 77: 541.

8. Schottenfield, D. and Fraumeni, J. F., Jr. (1982) Smoking and Drinking in relation to oral and pharyngeal cancers. Department of Health and Human Services, Washington D.C.

9. Seabright, M. (1971): A rapid banding technique for human chromosomes. Lancet II: 971.

10. Simarak, S., De Jong, U.W., Breslow, N. et al (1977): Cancer of the oral cavity, pharynx, larynx and lungin North Thailand. Case control study and analysis of cigar smoke. British Journal of Cancer 36: 130.

11. Sumner, A. T. (1972): A simple technique for demonstrating centromeric heterochromatin. Experimental Cell Research 75:304.

12. Tough, I. M., Buckton, K. E., Baikie, A. G. and Court-Brown, W. M. (1960): X-ray induced chromosome damage in man. Lancet II (7155): 849.

13. Vinnikov, V. A., Maznyk, N. A. and Lloyd, D. (2010): Delayed chromosomal instability in lymphocytes of cancer patients after radiotherapy. Int J Radiat Biol Apr; 86(4): 271-82.

14. Wahi, P.N., Luthra, U.K., Mali, S. and Shuinkin, N.B. (1972): Prevalance and distribution of cancer of the uterine cervix in Agra District, India. Cancer 30(3).

15. Wakefield, J., Yule, R., Smith, A. et al (1973): Relation of abnormal cytological smears and carcinoma of cervix uteri to

husband's occupation. British Medical Journal2: 142.

16. Warren, S. and Meisner, L. (1965): Chromosomal changes in

    leukocytes of patients receiving irradiation therapy. Journal of

    the American Medical Association 193(5): 351.

17. Wynder, E.L. and Stellman, S.D. (1977): Comparative

    epidemiology of tobacco-related cancer. Cancer Research 37:

    4608.

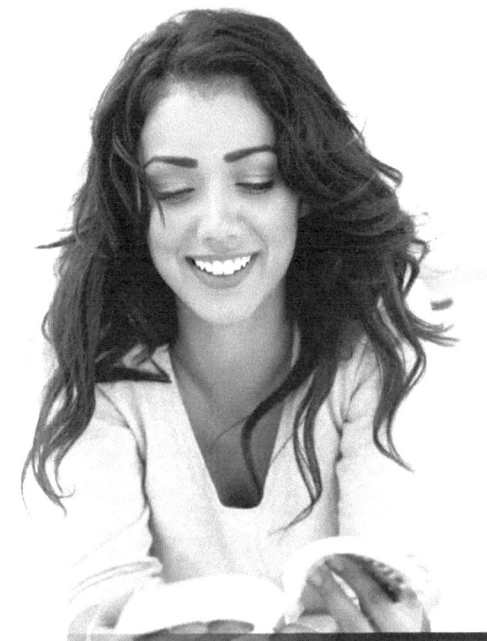
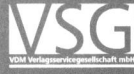

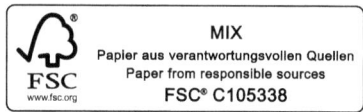